ENDOMETRIOSIS DIET BOOK

Special Meal Plan For Endometriosis Patients

CAMILLA REDDING

Table of Contents

CHAPTER 1

Endometriosis diet

Cells that resemble the uterine lining but are not cancerous, known as endometrial cells, proliferate outside of the uterus in endometriosis, which is a long-term condition. The endometrium is the lining of the uterus. The condition's name is derived from this.

According to the Endometriosis Foundation of America, one in ten American women will experience symptoms of the disease at some point in their reproductive lives.

Endometriosis is a condition that primarily affects women's reproductive organs. The spread of this tissue beyond the fallopian tubes, ovaries, and tissues lining the pelvic area is rare, but not impossible.

During menstruation, the symptoms of this condition tend

to be more pronounced. Among the symptoms:

Pain in the lower abdomen

• heightened discomfort during menstruation and intercourse

• Constipation and urination discomfort

Bleeding between periods that is too heavy or prolonged

• fatigue

• diarrhea

* bloating

* constipation

* Lower back ache

* a severe case of cramps

Endometriosis can cause infertility if left untreated.

People with a history of endometriosis have a slightly elevated risk of developing ovarian cancer or adenocarcinoma. The risk, according to The LancetTrusted Source, is still low over the course of a lifetime and treatment doesn't need to be rushed.

Currently, there is no cure for this condition, but it can be effectively managed with a multi-faceted approach. In order to get the best care, it's important to incorporate both a pain management plan and an exercise and nutrition regimen.

If you have endometriosis, keep reading to learn more about how your diet can help.

Nutrition plays a significant role in the development of endometriosis.

Few studies have examined the link between diet and symptoms of endometriosis. While some people find that certain foods cause or alleviate their symptoms, this isn't always the case.

Those who ate more vegetables and omega-3 fatty acids may have been better protected from endometriosis symptoms than those who ate more red meat, trans fats and coffee, according to a 2013 study. However, these findings vary from study to study, indicating that further investigation is required.

Endometriosis may be prevented or even worsened by eating a healthy diet, according to a study published in Brazil in 2015. Among the foods on this diet:

• fruits

• vegetables

The term "whole grains" refers to those that are

in addition to omega-3 fatty acids.

Endometriosis cannot be prevented, but according to the Office on Women's HealthTrusted Source, avoiding foods and chemicals that raise estrogen levels can reduce one's risk of developing it. Caffeine and alcohol are examples of these substances.

Dietary and lifestyle changes will not cure endometriosis, but they may help alleviate its symptoms.

A person with endometriosis may want to keep a food journal to see if their symptoms are affected by what they eat. They must keep track of everything they eat and any symptoms they experience throughout the day.

Keeping a diary may take some time, as a clear pattern may not become apparent right away.

What role does food play in the development of endometriosis?

CHAPTER 2

Endometriosis is a disease of the uterus.

Endometriosis symptoms can be exacerbated by inflammation and elevated estrogen levels. Both factors can be influenced by your diet.

To counteract inflammation and regulate estrogen, "food is essential," says Barth.. Endometriosis symptoms can be significantly reduced with the right diet, according to many people.

Fiber helps flush out excess estrogen.

Estrogen is a vital hormone, and it's necessary for normal bodily functions to have some of it. Endometriosis symptoms like cramping and pain can worsen if estrogen levels are too high.

Fortunately, this is where food and fiber come in handy.

"Excess estrogen is flushed out of your body through your bowel movements," says Barth. A regular bowel movement is essential to good health. If you don't, you may be suffering from constipation and/or excessive estrogen levels.

Get rid of constipation and excess estrogen by consuming a lot of fiber. Adults should consume 35 grams of fiber per day, according to Barth.

In order to get more fiber, simply eat more.

Eat the whole food, not just the juice.

• Grinded flaxseed, which can be used in smoothies or baked goods.

• Beans, lentils, and chickpeas, to name a few.

• Vegetables.

• Whole grains, such as brown rice and whole-wheat pasta.

Remember to gradually increase your fiber intake as you go along. Add a lot of fiber at once, and you'll experience gas and bloating. Avoid these side effects by gradually increasing your fiber intake and drinking plenty of water" Because of the high fiber content of ground flaxseed, no more than three tablespoons should be consumed per day.

Anti-inflammatory fats.

Inflammation exacerbates the symptoms of endometriosis, which is a chronic inflammatory disease. Endometriosis-related inflammation can be reduced by taking omega-3 fats. The following foods are high in omega-3 fatty acids:

Salmon, sardines, and tuna are examples of fatty fish.

Walnuts, chia seeds, and flaxseed are just a few of the many healthy nuts and seeds you can eat.

Flaxseed and canola oil are examples of plant oils.

Additionally, monounsaturated fats have the ability to reduce inflammation. In the following places can be found:

• Avocadoes.

• Seeds and nuts.

• Olive oil.

• Peanut butter. —

Oil made from safflower seeds.

Minerals that aid in muscle relaxation and menstrual cycle regulation

Calcium is a mineral that receives a lot of attention. Endometriosis sufferers, however, should supplement their magnesium and zinc intake.

In Barth's opinion, magnesium can help alleviate menstrual cramps. Natural muscle relaxant, that's what it is. The following foods are high in magnesium:

• Dark chocolate (but stick to small amounts, as it usually contains added sugar).

Greens such as kale and spinach, as well as arugula.

• Edamame and black beans, for instance.

• Almonds and pumpkin seeds, in particular.

For hormonal balance, zinc regulates your menstrual cycles. Barth explains that zinc aids in ovulation, or the release of an egg. You produce progesterone during ovulation, which counteracts estrogen. If you want to get pregnant, you'll need to ovulate.

Animal sources provide the most zinc. Ask your doctor if you should take a zinc supplement if you are vegetarian or vegan. Zinc can be found in these foods:

Chicken and turkey are examples of poultry.

• Consume two low-fat servings of red meat per week.

• Oysters, crab, and lobster are examples of shellfish.

CHAPTER 3

Endometriosis may be exacerbated by certain foods.

It is possible to increase your risk of developing endometriosis by making certain lifestyle choices. A person's ability to cope with or avoid the symptoms of a disorder may improve or worsen based on the decisions they make.

This condition may be exacerbated or even exacerbated by the following factors, although more research is needed to determine the exact relationship between them and endometriosis:

• A trans fat-rich diet. Women who consume more trans fat are more likely to be diagnosed with endometriosis, according to a study. Fried, processed, and fast food are the most common sources of trans fat. Find out why trans fats are so dangerous.

• Consumption of red meat. Red meat consumption has been linked to an increased risk of developing endometriosis, according to some studies.

• Gluten. After eliminating gluten from the diet, 75 percent of women with endometriosis reported a decrease in pain.

• Foods high in FODMAPs. Those with irritable bowel syndrome (IBS) and endometriosis who followed a low-FODMAP diet saw significant improvements in their symptoms, according to one study.

Endometriosis sufferers should avoid foods that affect hormone regulation, particularly estrogen balance. When it comes to reducing inflammation in the body, it is important to avoid or limit foods that may do so. A few examples include:

- alcohol

- caffeine

- gluten

- fatty meats

Saturated and trans fatty acids

Endometriosis-beneficial food sources

A nutrient-dense, well-balanced diet rich in plant-based foods and vitamins and minerals is the best way to combat the inflammation and pain caused by endometriosis. Dietary supplements:

Vegetables and fruits with a high fiber content (such as leafy greens and legumes)

Iron-rich foods such as dark greens, broccoli and beans;

fortified grains and cereals; as well as nut and seed products.

Salmon, sardines, herring, trout, walnuts, chia seeds, and flax seeds are good sources of essential fatty acids.

• Foods high in antioxidants, such as oranges, berries, dark chocolate, spinach, and beets;

If you eat certain foods, pay attention to how your body responds. Keeping a food diary and noting down your symptoms and triggers can be beneficial.

You might want to talk to a registered dietitian about your situation. There is no one-size-fits-all approach when it comes to food and endometriosis, so they can help you figure out what works best for you.

Is gluten or dairy linked to an increased risk of endometriosis?

Endometriosis sufferers may find relief from their symptoms by avoiding gluten and dairy products. In the end, it's up to the individual.

"Cutting out gluten or dairy is often the next step if you've tried eating healthier and it isn't enough," says Barth. At least a month of going gluten-free or dairy-free is usually recommended by me." If your symptoms return, gradually reintroduce it into your diet and monitor the results."

An additional benefit of the low-FODMAP diet is the ability to pinpoint problematic foods. If you suffer from IBS, the low-FODMAP diet can help, says Barth. Endometriosis sufferers can also benefit from the diet. It is possible that certain foods may exacerbate your endometriosis symptoms if you follow this diet closely.

Instead of making dietary changes, it's easy to reach for a bottle of pills. However, you shouldn't try supplements for endometriosis without first getting permission from your doctor.

In order to determine if you are deficient in any nutrients, your doctor can perform tests, as Barth explains. You can also take supplements if your doctor tells you to do so. If you're looking for a supplement that's right for you, don't go with the "one size fits all" approach."

Endometriosis weight loss plans

Look no further for endometriosis-friendly food options! Try out these recipes: "

At the beginning of the day, a dairy-free breakfast packed with fiber and healthy fat is a great way to get your day started. Make yourself a tropical breakfast bowl and see what you think.

It's a great lunch option because it's high in fiber and anti-inflammatory fats.

The healthy fats in baked fish and the fiber-rich vegetables make for a filling dinner.

If you're looking for something to nibble on between meals, this granola recipe is a great option. Nuts and seeds, which are rich in vitamins and minerals, make up the bulk of this dish.

Food has the power to heal the body and mind.

One of the best ways to manage endometriosis may be right in your own kitchen. "Change your diet if endometriosis interferes with your life," says Barth. You have nothing to lose, and you could gain a lot.

CHAPTER 4

Supplements that may be beneficial

As well as eating a nutritious diet, taking supplements may be beneficial as well.

A single, small study

At Trusted Source, 59 women with endometriosis participated in a study. Participants received 1,200 IU of vitamin E and 1,000 IU of vitamin C as dietary supplements. A decrease in inflammation and a decrease in chronic pelvic pain were observed in the study participants. These foods are rich in vitamin E and can help you get more of it in your diet.

Yet another investigation

Recommended dietary supplements from the aforementioned Trusted Source included zinc and the trio of vitamins A, C and E. Taking these supplements reduced peripheral oxidative stress and increased antioxidant markers in women with endometriosis.

Endometriosis management may also benefit from curcumin. Turmeric's anti-inflammatory component is found here. Curcumin reduced the production of estradiol, which inhibited endometrial cells, according to a study. Additionally, turmeric and curcumin have a slew of other health advantages.

Large-scale research project

According to Trusted Source, women with higher vitamin D levels and a higher dairy intake were less likely to have an increased risk of developing endometriosis. Calcium and magnesium, whether in food or supplement form, may be beneficial in addition to vitamin D.

Alternate methods of treatment and physical activity

Even endometriosis sufferers may benefit from regular exercise to manage their condition. Getting your heart rate up and your blood sugar up are two of the many benefits of working out.

Women with endometriosis may benefit from alternative therapies in addition to conventional treatments. A good example of this is the use of relaxation techniques. These could include, but are not limited to:

* meditation

* yoga

* acupuncture

* massage

Preventing endometriosis pain during sex is an important consideration for women with the condition.

A condition known as endometriosis is caused by the growth of cells in the ovaries, fallopian tubes, or bowel that are similar to those that line the uterus. These growths can cause sex to be painful at times.

Heavy menstrual bleeding, painful periods, and pain during sex are all signs of endometriosis.

In the medical community, sex-related pain is referred to as dyspareunia. In women with endometriosis, it is common because of the potential for stretching and pulling the endometrial growths during penetration and other sexual movements.

Endometriosis can cause painful sex in a variety of ways, which we explore in this article. In addition, we go over ways to deal with the pain, such as different positions, toys, and times, as well as how to talk about it with a partner.

Endometriosis can make sex painful for a variety of reasons.

Endometriosis can cause pain during sex, which is a common symptom. Endometrial tissue can be pulled and stretched by penetration and other movements during intercourse. This is especially true if endometrial tissue has grown behind the vagina or lower uterus.

This pain can also be caused by vaginal dryness. A hysterectomy (surgical removal of the uterus) or hormonal treatment for endometriosis can cause dryness.

Endometriosis does not cause pain in all women, however.

Those who do so run the risk of:

pain that comes on suddenly or as if it is stabbing

discomfort in the lower abdomen

• varying degrees of discomfort

A person's level of pain may vary depending on the type of intercourse they are involved in. Some people only feel pain during or after sex, while others feel pain both during and after sex.

Endometriosis-friendly positions

In some positions, endometrial tissue is less likely to be damaged. Experiment with your partner to find the best position for both of you.

However, some people prefer to work in certain positions. So, if you're on top, you can control the depth and speed of penetration, which gives you a more comfortable pace.

As a result, many comfortable positions necessitate only a shallow penetration. The following are a few examples of possible job duties:

• spooning

• Raising the endometriosis sufferer's hips

modifiable canine hairstyle

Women with endometriosis may find the missionary position difficult.

Penetrative sex can be painful for some people, so they may prefer other forms of sexual activity, such as:

The stimulation of the oral cavity

• massage

• foreplay

• playing with children's toys.

THE END